Narcissistic Mothers: The Truth about Being a Daughter of a Narcissistic Mother, and How to Overcome It. A Guide to Healing and Recovering from Narcissistic Abuse.

Alexandria Publications

Published by Digital Mind, 2024.

While every precaution has been taken in the preparation of this book, the publisher assumes no responsibility for errors or omissions, or for damages resulting from the use of the information contained herein.

NARCISSISTIC MOTHERS: THE TRUTH ABOUT BEING A DAUGHTER OF A NARCISSISTIC MOTHER, AND HOW TO OVERCOME IT. A GUIDE TO HEALING AND RECOVERING FROM NARCISSISTIC ABUSE.

First edition. February 4, 2024.

Copyright © 2024 Alexandria Publications.

ISBN: 979-8224094882

Written by Alexandria Publications.

Also by Alexandria Publications

Table of Contents

Introduction 1

Chapter 1: Narcissistic Mothers 3

Chapter 2: Roots of Maternal Narcissism 11

Chapter 3: Effects on Children 19

Chapter 4: Cycles of Emotional Abuse from the book narcissistic mothers 25

Chapter 5: Coping Strategies 31

Chapter 6: The Road to Recovery 37

Chapter 7: Therapy and Support Resources 43

Chapter 8: Adult Mother-Child Relationships 49

Chapter 9: Impact on Parenting 55

Chapter 10: Case Studies and Testimonials 61

Conclusion 65

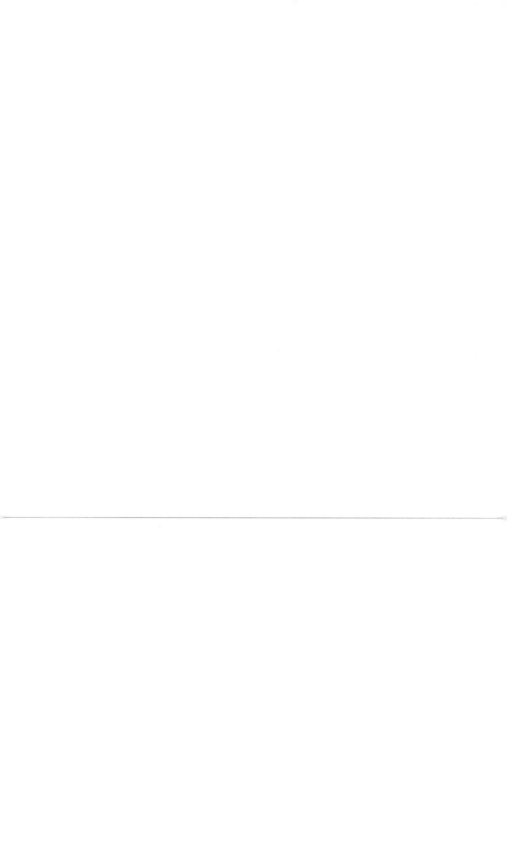

Introduction

In the vast spectrum of human relationships, the mother-child connection stands as a foundation, an emotional support network meant to nourish and flourish. However, in the complicated web of these relationships, an intriguing and challenging psychological phenomenon sometimes reveals itself: maternal narcissism.

But what does it really mean to be a narcissistic mother? Simplifying the idea, we are referring to those mothers whose main focus seems to be their own image and desires, overshadowing, often without realizing it, the emotional needs of their own children. This book seeks to delve into this phenomenon, shedding light on a dark and little explored corner of maternal psychology.

To understand this complex phenomenon, let's imagine an emotional theater where narcissistic mothers play the main role. On the public stage, they may project an impeccable image of motherhood, but behind the scenes, the masks slip, revealing a complexity of emotions and behaviors. These mothers are like skilled actresses who masterfully change their masks depending on the circumstances, leaving their children trapped in a confusing dance of identity.

In childhood, a crucial period for the formation of the being, these mothers plant seeds in the fertile soil of the child's psyche. The mother's constant overvaluation and lack of validation for the child's individual experiences can become an emotional storm that affects the child's self-image and self-esteem.

It is essential to recognize that talking about maternal narcissism is not an act of rebellion, but rather a courageous step toward understanding and healing. Many who have grown up in the shadow of narcissistic mothers carry invisible emotional scars, marked by the innate desire to be seen and validated. Breaking the silence around these painful experiences is the first step towards emotional release.

On this journey of exploration, we will address the complexities of maternal narcissism without complicated jargon or inaccessible psychological terms. We seek to build a bridge between specialized research and everyday understanding, allowing both those familiar with psychology and those who are not, to immerse themselves in the plot of this human story.

Throughout these pages, we will delve into the cycles of emotional abuse, explore coping strategies, and reflect on the possibility of healing and growth. This book is not only an attempt to decipher the riddle of narcissistic mothers, but also a beacon of hope for those seeking to understand, accept, and ultimately break free from the emotional chains that may have marked their past.

In every word written, we aim to provide a map that guides readers through this complex terrain and, in doing so, offer a space where empathy and understanding can flourish. Ultimately, this book is a testament to human strength, resilience , and the ability to find light even in the darkest places of our emotional experiences.

Chapter 1: Narcissistic Mothers

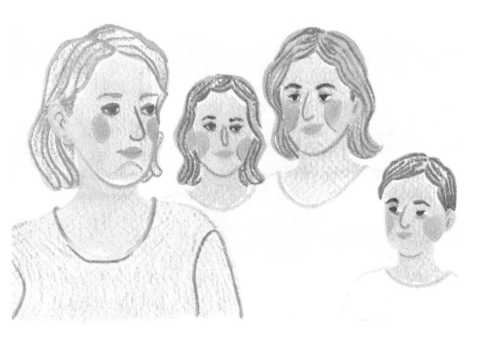

On this journey of psychological exploration, we enter complex emotional territory: the world of narcissistic mothers. For many, the term "narcissism" conjures images of vanity and self-centeredness, but in the context of motherhood, this phenomenon takes on a unique and challenging dimension. In this first chapter, we will dive into the turbulent waters of mother-child relationships marked by narcissism, seeking to understand the roots, impacts and mysteries of this emotional enigma.

Imagine, if you can, the concept of a mother whose universe revolves intensely around her self-image, her desires, and her achievements. This mother, who could be such an essential figure in a child's life, often finds herself caught in a complicated dance of unmet emotional needs. Thus, we enter the territory of narcissistic mothers, women whose way of approaching motherhood is marked by a constant search for validation and attention.

1.1 Definition and characteristics of maternal narcissism Beginning of the form

Simplified Definition of Maternal Narcissism

In simple terms, maternal narcissism refers to a pattern of behavior in which the mother focuses her attention disproportionately on herself, her needs and desires, often overshadowing the emotional needs of her own children. This excessive focus on the self can manifest in various ways in the mother-child dynamic and can have a significant impact on the emotional development of children.

Imagine a mother viewing her children through the prism of her own existence, evaluating them by how well they reflect her self-image and satisfy her emotional needs. This mother may constantly seek external validation, seeking for her children to fill the emotional void that she herself may not have been able to fill.

Key Characteristics of Maternal Narcissism

Now that we have established a basic definition, let's explore some of the key characteristics that outline maternal narcissism.

1. **Constant Overvaluation:** A narcissistic mother can overvalue her children in an apparently positive way. However, this overvaluation can be exaggerated and conditional, linked to the child's ability to satisfy the mother's emotional needs. The child's achievements become an extension of the mother's ego, rather than individual celebrations of the child's growth and success.

2. **Lack of Empathy:** Empathy, that ability to put yourself in someone else's shoes, is often diminished in a narcissistic mother. The children's experiences and emotions may be minimized or ignored, as the mother's attention is strongly focused on her own concerns and desires.

3. **Emotional Masks:** On the public stage, the narcissistic mother can project an image of impeccable motherhood, receiving praise and admiration from those around her. However, in the privacy of the home, the masks slip,

revealing the complexity and sometimes darkness of the mother's true feelings and behaviors.

4. **Emotional Manipulation:** Emotional manipulation can be a common tool in a narcissistic mother's arsenal. This can manifest itself through subtly coercive tactics aimed at controlling the children's emotions and actions to satisfy the mother's needs.

5. **Constantly Seeks Validation:** The narcissistic mother continually seeks external validation to maintain her self-image. This search can extend to the relationship with their children, who often find themselves in the role of providers of that validation, generating an unequal dynamic in the relationship.

6. **Unrealistic Expectations:** The narcissistic mother's expectations can be excessive and unrealistic. She expects her children to meet high standards, and at the same time, she hopes those achievements will reflect positively on her.

7. **Difficulty Accepting Criticism:** Criticism, even constructive, can be poorly received by a narcissistic mother. The fragility of her self-image may cause her to reject any suggestion that there might be areas for improvement in her maternal approach.

Understanding these characteristics provides a framework for exploring the complexities of relationships affected by maternal narcissism. Each of these facets contributes to a unique dynamic that can have significant consequences on the emotional development of children.

It is essential to remember that, although these characteristics outline patterns of behavior observed in narcissistic mothers, not all mothers who exhibit some of these characteristics are automatically classified as narcissistic. The complexity of human relationships involves a variety of factors, and each situation is unique.

1.2 Impact on the lives of children

A) Emotional Development and Self-Esteem

One of the most significant impacts is the influence on the emotional development of children. Imagine an emotional garden where self-esteem and self-confidence should flourish. With a narcissistic mother, this garden can be affected by a persistent shadow. Children may grow up feeling that their worth is directly linked to the ability to meet their mother's emotional needs.

Self-esteem, that internal assessment of oneself, can falter under the weight of unrealistic expectations and a lack of genuine validation. Children may internalize the idea that they are never good enough, since the narcissistic mother's attention and affection are given conditionally, based on meeting her expectations.

B) Interpersonal Relationships

The impact extends beyond the mother-child relationship, affecting the way children relate to others. Growing up with a narcissistic mother can influence your ability to form healthy, meaningful relationships. A lack of empathy and a self-centered approach can make it difficult for children to understand and connect emotionally with others.

The constant search for validation can lead to behavioral patterns in which children excessively seek external approval, creating unbalanced interpersonal dynamics. They may become extremely sensitive to criticism and have difficulty setting healthy boundaries in their relationships.

C) Anxiety and Depression

The emotional weight of growing up with a narcissistic mother can lead to mental health problems, such as anxiety and depression. The constant pressure to meet unrealistic expectations and a lack of emotional support can lead to high levels of stress. Children may feel trapped in a cycle of constantly seeking approval, accompanied by anxiety about not being able to meet maternal expectations.

Lack of validation and recognition of your own emotional needs can contribute to feelings of sadness and hopelessness. Children may experience the feeling that their achievements are not good enough, regardless of the effort invested, which can fuel depression.

D) Identity Development

The process of personal identity formation is also influenced by the presence of a narcissistic mother. Children may struggle to develop a strong, positive understanding of who they really are as their experiences are overshadowed by the mother's needs and desires.

Instead of encouraging individual exploration and expression, a narcissistic mother may impose her own expectations and desires on her children, limiting their ability to discover and embrace their unique identity. This can create a feeling of confusion and disconnection from oneself.

E) Fear of Abandonment and Codependent Relationships

The dynamic with a narcissistic mother can sow seeds of fear of abandonment. Children may learn to fear the loss of maternal approval and, therefore, may develop codependent behavior patterns . This can manifest itself in constantly seeking the approval of others, often sacrificing one's own needs in the process.

Emotional dependency can become a survival strategy, as children learn to adapt to the changing demands of the narcissistic mother to maintain an illusory sense of connection and security.

1.3 Recognizing patterns of narcissistic behavior

For those who have grown up with a narcissistic mother, recognizing specific behavioral patterns can be a critical but challenging task. It is not just about understanding the general characteristics of maternal narcissism, but rather identifying how these characteristics manifest themselves in everyday life.

1. Constant Need for Attention and Validation

One of the most obvious patterns is the constant need for attention and validation from the mother. Imagine a scenario where all conversations, decisions and achievements must focus on her. If you notice that your mother always directs the conversation toward herself, constantly seeks praise, and needs to be in the center of attention, these could be signs of a narcissistic dynamic.

This pattern may be especially evident in situations where it should be a special time for the child, such as graduations, personal achievements, or important events. If your mother tends to make these moments about her, seeking praise and downplaying your accomplishments, you may be dealing with a narcissistic mother.

2. Lack of Empathy and Emotional Understanding

Lack of empathy is another key characteristic. Try to remember situations in which you shared your feelings or worries with your mother. Did she show genuine understanding and emotional support, or did she steer the conversation toward her own experiences and emotions? A narcissistic mother often finds it difficult to connect emotionally with others as her own needs and emotions come to the fore.

This pattern can manifest itself in a variety of ways, from minimizing your feelings to completely ignoring your emotional experiences. A lack of empathy can create an environment where you feel misunderstood and emotionally disconnected from your mother.

3. Subtle Manipulation to Get What You Want

Subtle manipulation is a common tactic in a narcissistic mother's repertoire. It can manifest itself in a variety of ways, from using tears to gain sympathy to applying blame to get you to meet their expectations. If you notice that your mother has a talent for making you feel responsible for her happiness or that she uses manipulative tactics to get what she wants, you could be dealing with narcissistic behavior.

Manipulation can also appear in the form of criticism disguised as well-intentioned advice. A narcissistic mother may use seemingly constructive feedback to subtly control your choices and actions.

4. Anger or Anger in the Face of Contradiction

Another pattern to take into account is your mother's reaction to the contradiction. Narcissistic mothers may have difficulty accepting divergent or critical opinions. If you notice that your mother reacts with anger, irritation, or even contempt when you disagree with her, this could be an indication of a narcissistic pattern.

This behavior can make you feel self-conscious about expressing your own opinions, contributing to a dynamic where your mother dictates the narrative and you are forced to conform to her perspectives.

5. Constant Competition and Unfavorable Comparisons

The narcissistic mother often views her children as an extension of herself. If you notice constant competition or unfavorable comparisons between you and your siblings or other people, this may be a clear sign. The narcissistic mother may perceive her children as a threat to her own image, generating a dynamic in which she seeks to maintain control and superiority.

This pattern can significantly affect your self-esteem and contribute to the feeling of never being good enough, as unfavorable comparisons create an impossible standard to achieve.

6. Change of Attitude towards Constructive Criticism

Observe how your mother reacts to constructive criticism. A healthy mother can accept feedback aimed at improving the relationship and addressing problems. On the other hand, a narcissistic mother may reject any suggestion for improvement, interpreting it as a personal attack.

If you notice that your mother has difficulty receiving constructive criticism and always reacts with defense or denial, this could be indicative of a narcissistic pattern.

7. Use of Guilt as a Control Tool

The narcissistic mother can use guilt as an effective control tool. If you feel that your mother has the ability to make you feel responsible for her happiness or that she uses blaming tactics to get what she wants, you are observing a narcissistic pattern.

This behavior can create a sense of obligation and emotional responsibility toward your mother, creating a dynamic in which you feel trapped and obligated to meet her needs at the expense of your own.

Recognizing these patterns of narcissistic behavior is not an exercise in finger-pointing, but rather a tool for understanding the underlying dynamics in the mother-child relationship. Identifying these signs can be the first step toward understanding and eventually building healthy boundaries and effective coping strategies.

Chapter 2: Roots of Maternal Narcissism

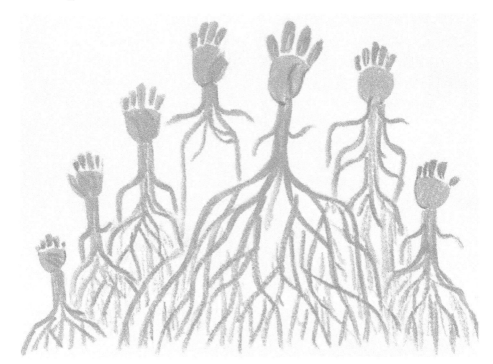

Understanding the roots of maternal narcissism involves looking beyond the superficial manifestations of behavior. It is not simply a matter of identifying the obvious characteristics, but of delving into the psychological terrain where these dynamics originate and take shape. In doing so, we not only illuminate the factors that contribute to maternal narcissism, but we also cultivate a deeper understanding of mothers who exhibit these patterns and how these characteristics affect relationships with their children.

Maternal narcissism, at its core, is a complex manifestation of the human psyche, influenced by an intersection of biological, psychological, and environmental factors. Exploring the roots of this phenomenon involves considering various perspectives and examining the interaction of these factors in personality development and parenting dynamics.

2.1 Psychological and environmental factors

To truly understand the roots of maternal narcissism, we must delve into the intricate nuances of the psychological and environmental factors that shape this complex dynamic.

Psychological Factors: Exploring the Depths of Personality

From a psychological perspective, maternal narcissism finds its roots in the complexity of personality and how certain traits develop over time. Two prominent psychological theories, Freud's psychoanalytic theory and Bowlby 's attachment theory , offer valuable perspectives on how psychological factors contribute to maternal narcissism.

According to Freud, narcissism originates in an early phase of psychosexual development, where the child experiences self-centered pleasure. If this phase is not completed adequately, the individual may develop a narcissistic orientation in which the search for gratification is centered on the self. In the context of maternal narcissism, a mother who does not adequately facilitate her child's transition toward a more external orientation may contribute to the formation of narcissistic characteristics.

Bowlby 's attachment theory , on the other hand, highlights the importance of early relationships, especially the relationship between mother and child, in the formation of personality. If the mother is unable to provide a secure attachment environment and emotional nourishment, the child may develop insecure attachment patterns which, in turn, contribute to the development of narcissistic characteristics.

Environmental Factors: The Role of the Environment in the Formation of Maternal Narcissism

In environments that disproportionately emphasize performance, appearance, and external validation, children may internalize these values and develop a narcissistic orientation. If a mother overvalues social status, material success, or appearance, these values can be passed on to her children, influencing their search for validation and recognition.

Family dynamics and social interactions also play a crucial role. A child who grows up in an environment where attention and validation are scarce may develop coping strategies that align with narcissistic patterns to seek missing attention. In these situations, narcissism can arise as a response to the constant need to feel valued.

Influence of Stress and Trauma: How Difficult Experiences Contribute to Maternal Narcissism

Stress and trauma are factors that should not be underestimated when exploring the roots of maternal narcissism. Traumatic experiences, whether in a mother's childhood or throughout her life, can have a significant impact on the way she approaches motherhood.

Narcissism can become a defense mechanism against stress or emotional pain, creating a barrier that makes it difficult to emotionally connect with your children. Instead of facing the pain, the mother may take refuge in narcissistic behaviors as a way to protect herself emotionally.

Cultural and Social Influences: The Broader Context of the Formation of Maternal Narcissism

Maternal narcissism is also influenced by the cultural and social norms surrounding a community. Societies that overvalue individualism, material success, and competition can encourage the emergence of narcissistic characteristics in parenting.

Cultural expectations about the role of the mother and pressures to meet socially imposed standards may contribute to the formation of maternal narcissism. In a context where external validation is considered crucial, mothers may internalize these expectations and pass them on to their children.

These factors do not exist in isolation; rather, they interact in complex and multifaceted ways, creating the breeding ground for the development of narcissistic behaviors in motherhood.

2.2 Genetic inheritance and its influence

1. What Does Genetic Inheritance Mean in the Context of Maternal Narcissism?

When we talk about genetic inheritance in the context of maternal narcissism, we are referring to the transmission of certain traits and predispositions through genes from one generation to another. Genes are like instructions encoded in our DNA that influence various aspects of our personality, behavior and, yes, even the way mothers relate to their children.

It is crucial to emphasize from the beginning that genetic inheritance is not an immutable destiny. We are not irrevocably tied to inherited traits. Rather, the interaction between genetics and environment plays a critical role in the expression of these traits. Therefore, when we talk about the influence of genetic inheritance on maternal narcissism, we are exploring how certain narcissistic traits may have a genetic basis, but also how these traits develop and are expressed in the context of upbringing and childhood experiences. life.

2. Genetic Traits Associated with Maternal Narcissism: What Does the Research Say?

Research in the field of psychology and genetics has shed light on certain traits and predispositions that may have a connection to maternal narcissism. However, it is essential to approach this with the understanding that genetics does not operate in a simple and direct way. The relationship between genetics and behavior is complex and multifaceted.

Some studies suggest that genetic predisposition may contribute to vulnerability to developing narcissistic traits. These traits may include a greater need for external validation, a tendency to seek praise, and an orientation toward the self in social interaction. However, it is crucial to remember that the expression of these traits can be strongly influenced by upbringing and life experiences.

3. How Genetic and Environmental Interaction Develops: An Intricate Dance

The interaction between genes and environment is like an intricate dance in which each influences the other constantly. In the case of maternal narcissism, genes can establish certain predispositions, but it is the environment that activates, modulates and shapes the expression of these traits.

Imagine genes as a set of instructions. These instructions may be present in our DNA from birth, but their activation and expression depend largely on life experiences and environmental interactions. A mother with genetic predispositions toward narcissistic traits may or may not develop these traits depending on her environment and parenting experiences.

4. The Role of Parenting and Life Experiences: Modeling Maternal Narcissism

Upbringing and life experiences are like sculptors that shape the expression of genetic traits. A mother with genetic predispositions toward narcissism may manifest or mitigate these traits depending on the quality of her relationship with her own parents, her social environment, and the life experiences she has gone through.

For example, a mother who has experienced nurturing parenting and developed stress management skills may be less likely to express narcissistic traits, even if she has genetic predispositions toward them. On the other hand, a mother with the same genetic predispositions, but who has faced traumatic life experiences or emotional shortcomings, may manifest these narcissistic traits more pronounced.

5. The Importance of Awareness and Self-Exploration

Genetic inheritance in the context of maternal narcissism urges us to reflect on the importance of awareness and self-exploration. Being aware of our own genetic predispositions and being open to exploring our life experiences can be crucial steps toward understanding how they influence how we relate to our children.

Self-exploration also allows us to be active agents in shaping our own parenting interactions. Recognizing inherited patterns and consciously working to change those that may be unhealthy is a powerful act of self-determination.

2.3 Development of narcissistic personality in the mother

A) Childhood and Early Childhood: The Initial Seeds of Personality

Personality development begins in the earliest stages of life. During infancy and early childhood, the mother experiences a crucial interaction with her environment and caregivers. The quality of these interactions influences the formation of their personality and establishes the foundation for future parenting dynamics.

If the mother experiences affectionate care, emotional support, and a secure relationship with her own parents, she is more likely to develop a balanced and empathetic personality. However, if these experiences are poor or traumatic, defense mechanisms may arise, including narcissistic traits.

B) Adolescence: The Search for Identity and Validation

Adolescence marks a crucial phase in personality development. During this period, the mother searches for her identity and strives to obtain external validation. If emotional needs are not adequately met during adolescence, narcissistic patterns may emerge as a strategy to gain attention and validation that may have been absent.

Social and cultural pressure also plays an important role during adolescence. If the mother lives in an environment that overvalues material success, appearance, or social status, she may internalize these values and develop a narcissistic orientation in seeking to meet these expectations.

C) Transition to Motherhood: The Influence of Previous Parenting Experience

The transition to motherhood is a crucial period that can intensify or mitigate a mother's narcissistic traits. Previous parenting experiences, especially the relationship with your own mother, have a significant impact. If the mother experienced warm parenting and healthy parenting models, she is more likely to adopt similar parenting patterns.

However, if previous parenting experiences were challenging or lacked emotional support, the mother may face difficulty establishing strong emotional connections with her own children. This is where narcissistic traits can manifest, as the mother may focus more on her own needs and desires than the needs of her children.

D) Stressful and Traumatic Factors: Triggers of Maternal Narcissism

Stressors and traumatic factors can act as significant triggers in the development of narcissistic personality in a mother. Experiences such as the loss of a loved one, financial problems, divorce or other stressful events can trigger the activation of narcissistic defense mechanisms as a way of coping with emotional pain.

The mother may turn to herself for comfort, neglecting the emotional needs of her children. This behavior can intensify if the mother lacks skills to manage stress in a healthy way.

E) Continuous Interaction with the Environment: Feedback from Narcissistic Traits

Throughout life, continuous interaction with the environment continues to influence the development of the narcissistic personality in the mother. Parenting experiences, personal and professional relationships, and social interactions remain formative factors. If the mother continually experiences situations that reinforce the importance of her own needs over those of others, narcissistic traits can persist and become stronger.

Chapter 3: Effects on Children

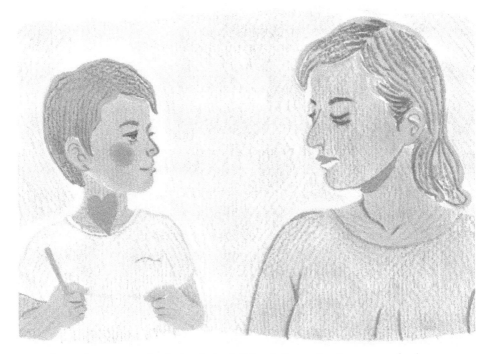

M others play a central role in their children's lives, shaping not only the way they perceive the world, but also how they perceive themselves. In this chapter we will appreciate the emotional traces left by maternal narcissism, exploring how these early experiences can influence the emotional, social and psychological development of children. From childhood to adolescence, we will unravel the complexities of mother-child relationships marked by narcissism, seeking to understand not only the what, but also the how, of these lasting effects. Through this analysis, we aim to shed light on the challenges and possibilities for healing, forging a path toward healthier, more equitable relationships.

3.1 How narcissism affects the emotional

development of children

The impact of maternal narcissism on the emotional development of children is complex and delicate territory that deserves detailed exploration. In this section, we delve into the shadows of emotional validation, examining how the presence of a mother with narcissistic tendencies can leave a deep mark on her children's internal world.

Gaps in Emotional Validation: The Echo of Unmet Needs

A narcissistic mother is often more focused on her own needs and desires than on the feelings and emotional needs of her children. This lack of emotional validation can create a persistent echo in the emotional development of children, leaving them with a feeling of invisibility and a constant struggle for recognition.

From expressions of joy to moments of sadness, children seek validation of their emotions as an essential component to building a solid emotional foundation. However, in the context of maternal narcissism, this validation may be lacking. Children may learn to suppress their emotions or doubt their own emotional worth, as their experiences are not validated or recognized by the narcissistic mother.

Impact on Self-Esteem: Seeds of Self-Doubt and Distrust

Self-esteem, that delicate sprout in a child's emotional garden, can be significantly affected by a lack of emotional validation. The narcissistic mother, focused on her own world, can leave her children with seeds of doubt and distrust in themselves.

The constant search for validation that characterizes childhood and adolescence can become a thorny path when the narcissistic mother does not offer the necessary emotional support. Children may begin to question their worth and tirelessly seek external approval, since internal validation has been diminished by the emotional lack in their relationship with their mother.

Difficulties in Managing Emotions: The Absence of Suitable Models

The mother is not only a figure of affection, but also a crucial model for the healthy management and expression of emotions. In the case of maternal narcissism, children may face difficulties in developing adequate emotional skills.

The narcissistic mother, focused on her own needs, may not provide a strong example of how to manage emotions constructively. This can result in children struggling to understand and express their own feelings, facing challenges in emotional regulation and building healthy relationships later in life.

Forming Fragile Emotional Bonds: The Shadow of the Disrupted Connection

Healthy emotional development is built on the foundation of strong emotional connections. The narcissistic mother, however, can contribute to the formation of fragile and distant emotional bonds with her children. Lack of emotional connection can lead to a feeling of loneliness and a constant search for affection and validation in other relationships.

Children may experience difficulties establishing secure and satisfying emotional relationships, as the narcissistic mother may not have provided the model of necessary emotional connection during childhood. The shadow of the interrupted connection can haunt children into their adult lives, affecting the quality of their relationships and their ability to form strong emotional bonds.

3.2 Family relationships and dysfunctional dynamics

Family relationships are the fabric that makes up the fabric of our lives, and when the shadow of maternal narcissism hangs over them, the dynamics can become complex and, in many cases, dysfunctional. In this segment, we will look at the shadows of disconnection that can color family relationships when a mother exhibits narcissistic tendencies.

1. Competition Instead of Collaboration: The Race for Validation

In families affected by maternal narcissism, collaboration can give way to competition, and external validation becomes a coveted resource. Children may feel that they must compete with each other for the attention and approval of the narcissistic mother, creating dynamics of rivalry rather than mutual support.

This competition can sow seeds of discord between siblings, generating tensions that persist throughout life. The shadow of rivalry can darken family relationships, making it difficult to build solid and healthy bonds between siblings.

2. The Role of the Scapegoat and the Favorite: Toxic Dynamics in the Narcissistic Family

In some families with a narcissistic mother, toxic dynamics can arise, such as the role of scapegoat and favorite. The narcissistic mother may project her own frustrations and unfulfilled desires onto one child, designating him or her as the scapegoat, while elevating another as the favorite.

This dynamic creates tensions and imbalances in family relationships. The scapegoat may feel constantly singled out and belittled, while the favorite may experience overwhelming pressure to meet the mother's expectations. The shadows of these dynamics can last into adult life, affecting children's self-esteem and relationships.

3. Lack of Autonomy Support: The Weight of Unrealistic Expectations

In a narcissistic environment, the mother may have unrealistic expectations about her children's role and achievements. It can be difficult for children to find support in autonomy and decision-making, as the narcissistic mother can impose her own aspirations and desires without considering individual needs.

This lack of support in the development of autonomy can have long-term consequences. Children may face difficulties making independent decisions, experiencing a feeling of lack of control over their own lives. The shadows of these dysfunctional dynamics can be projected into the children's personal and professional relationships.

4. Challenges in Building Healthy Relationships: The Shadow of Mistrust and Broken Intimacy

Narcissistic family relationships can sow the seeds of mistrust and broken intimacy in children. Lack of emotional validation and focus on the mother's needs can make it difficult to establish healthy, meaningful relationships in adult life.

Children may experience difficulty trusting others and forming deep emotional connections, as previous family experiences have left scars on their ability to trust and share openly.

5. Healing Family Dynamics: Strategies to Rebuild Connections

Despite the shadows of dysfunctional dynamics, healing and rebuilding family connections are possible. In the following sections of this chapter, we will explore specific strategies designed to address dysfunctional dynamics and foster healthier relationships.

From setting healthy boundaries to encouraging open communication, these strategies are designed to help children navigate the shadows of narcissistic family relationships and build stronger ground for meaningful, equitable connections in the future.

3.3 The role of narcissism in the formation of children's self-esteem

Children's self-esteem is a delicate bud that is nourished by the interactions, support and emotional validation that children receive from their parents. In the context of maternal narcissism, the mirror in which children seek to reflect themselves may be clouded.

A) Conditioned Validation: The Challenge of Being "Good" to Be Loved

In families affected by maternal narcissism, emotional validation can become conditional on meeting certain standards. Children may feel that their worth and love are directly linked to their ability to meet the expectations and needs of the narcissistic mother.

This conditioning can have a profound impact on the formation of self-esteem. Children may internalize the belief that they are only worthy of love and appreciation when they comply with their mother's demands, creating a fragile foundation for their self-concept .

B) The Broken Mirror: Distortions in Self-Perception

Self-esteem is nourished by the image that children have of themselves, but in the narcissistic environment, this mirror can fracture. The lack of validation and emotional support can lead to distortions in self-perception, where children may see unrealistic expectations and negative self-evaluations reflected.

The narcissistic mother, by focusing on her own needs, may not provide the clear, positive mirror that children need to build a healthy self-image. On the other hand, children may see unrealistic criticism and expectations reflected, generating doubts about their worth and abilities.

C) The Weight of Comparisons: Being the Mirror of the Mother's Unfulfilled Desires

In a narcissistic environment, children can become the reflection of the mother's unfulfilled desires. The narcissistic mother may project her own aspirations and expectations onto her children, comparing them to an idealized standard that may be unattainable.

This constant comparison can have a devastating impact on children's self-esteem. They may feel that they never meet the mother's expectations, leading to negative self-evaluation and the belief that they will never be good enough.

D) Impact on Emotional Resilience : The Shadow of Vulnerability

Childhood self-esteem is also intertwined with emotional resilience , the ability to face challenges and overcome adversity. In a narcissistic environment, the lack of emotional support can weaken the resilience of children.

The constant need to meet the narcissistic mother's expectations can lead to a feeling of vulnerability and fear of failure. Children may face difficulty developing the resilience necessary to face life's challenges as they have been conditioned to seek external validation as a measure of their worth.

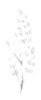

Chapter 4: Cycles of Emotional Abuse from the book narcissistic mothers

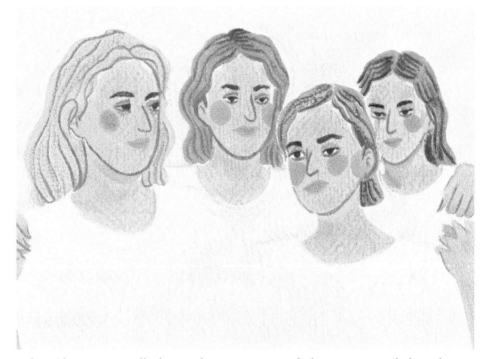

In this Chapter we will observe how narcissistic behavior is revealed in the waves of manipulation and silent pain that impact children. We will explore how these cycles of emotional abuse intertwine in mother-child relationships, leaving invisible but deep scars in the fabric of the child's psyche. As we navigate these turbulent waters, we will seek to understand the nature of these cycles, their lasting effects, and strategies to break the cycle and foster healing.

4.1 Repetitive patterns in mother-child interactions

In relationships affected by maternal narcissism, the repetitive patterns in mother-child interactions resemble waves that, instead of dissipating, persist, forming incessant cycles that deeply affect the children.

The Perpetual Search for Validation: A Constant Echo

At the heart of many repetitive patterns is the children's perpetual search for validation. The narcissistic mother, focused on her own needs, can establish a cycle where the children constantly seek approval and recognition of their worth. This cycle can become an exhausting dance, as children desperately seek to meet the mother's changing expectations to gain even a glimmer of validation.

These interactions can create a repetitive pattern where children feel like they never measure up, which in turn reinforces the constant search for validation. The cycle of searching, not finding, and searching again can leave children emotionally exhausted and feeling worthless.

Subtle Manipulation: When Waves Become Whirlwinds of Confusion

In relationships affected by maternal narcissism, subtle manipulation becomes a repetitive pattern that weaves an invisible but powerful thread into mother-child interactions. The narcissistic mother may use manipulative tactics to maintain control and ensure that the children meet her needs and expectations.

This manipulation can take various forms, from the use of blame to creating an environment where children feel they must constantly guess at the mother's changing needs. Children may find themselves trapped in a cycle of confusion and doubt as expectations are not clearly communicated, and any deviation can trigger intense emotional reactions on the part of the mother.

Cycles of Devaluation: When Waves Turn into Storms of Fragmented Self-Esteem

Devaluation cycles are a distinctive feature in mother-child interactions in the context of maternal narcissism. The narcissistic mother may establish a pattern where she consistently devalues her children's achievements and worth. This cycle can have a devastating impact on children's self-esteem, creating an environment where they never feel good enough.

Constant devaluation can lead children to internalize a sense of unworthiness and constantly question their own abilities and achievements. This repetitive pattern can leave deep scars on the psyche, affecting children's perception of themselves throughout life.

Unrealistic Expectations: Cycles of Unattainable Perfectionism

In relationships affected by maternal narcissism, cycles of unrealistic expectations become a repetitive pattern that can stifle the children's self-esteem and self-acceptance . The narcissistic mother may set impossibly high standards, creating a constant cycle of relentless efforts to meet unattainable expectations.

This repetitive pattern can lead to a persistent feeling of not measuring up and generate constant anxiety about not meeting the mother's expectations. Children may feel like they can never be perfect enough, which can negatively affect their self-concept and their ability to set healthy boundaries in future relationships.

Breaking the Cycles: Strategies to Address Repetitive Patterns

Despite the persistence of these repetitive patterns in mother-child interactions, it is crucial to highlight that there is the possibility of breaking these cycles and promoting healing. In the following sections of this chapter, we will explore specific strategies designed to address and modify these repetitive patterns.

From setting healthy boundaries to encouraging open communication, these strategies are designed to empower children and help them break free from cycles of manipulation and devaluation. By unraveling repetitive patterns, we aim to open a path to healthier, more equitable relationships.

4.2 Psychological abuse and emotional manipulation

Within relationships affected by maternal narcissism, psychological abuse and emotional manipulation can overshadow the mental and emotional health of children. We explore the intricate ways in which these patterns of abuse manifest, creating an environment where emotional wounds are deep yet invisible, and where pain is intertwined with the daily reality of children.

1. The Power Play: Manipulation to Maintain Control

The narcissistic mother often uses manipulation tactics to maintain control in the mother-child dynamic. This power play can manifest itself in a variety of ways, from subtle emotional manipulation to creating situations where children feel they must comply with the mother's changing expectations to avoid negative consequences.

Manipulation can create an insidious cycle where children find themselves trapped in the constant search to please their mother and avoid conflict. This pattern can leave children feeling helpless and trapped in an exhausting emotional cycle.

2. Attrition of Self-Esteem: Strategies to Undermine Children's Confidence

Psychological abuse often includes strategies aimed at undermining children's self-esteem. The narcissistic mother may use critical comments, constant devaluation, and unfavorable comparisons to erode the children's self-confidence.

These subtle but persistent attacks can have a significant impact on children's self-esteem and self-image. The constant repetition of negative messages can lead children to internalize a distorted perception of themselves, negatively affecting their emotional well-being over time.

3. Mind Games: Creating Confusion and Constant Doubts

Emotional manipulation often involves mind games designed to create constant confusion and doubt in the minds of children. The narcissistic mother can constantly change the rules of the game, creating an environment where the children feel that they can never predict the mother's reactions and expectations.

This pattern of mind games can leave children feeling constantly insecure and anxious. Lack of clarity and ambiguity in interactions can generate a persistent feeling of being on guard, contributing to emotional and psychological exhaustion.

4. Emotional Isolation: The Manipulation that Breaks Bonds

The narcissistic mother often uses emotional manipulation to isolate her children emotionally. It can create an environment where children feel that sharing their emotions and experiences is dangerous or not allowed. Manipulation can generate a cloak of emotional silence, where children are afraid to express their true feelings.

Emotional isolation can have lasting consequences on children's relationships, as they may face difficulties establishing healthy emotional connections in adult life. The shadow of manipulation that breaks ties can linger, affecting children's ability to trust and share in future relationships.

4.3 Long-term consequences for adult children

A) Lasting Emotional Wounds: The Weight of Childhood Marked by Narcissism

The emotional wounds inflicted during childhood under the influence of maternal narcissism do not fade with age. In adulthood, children can carry the weight of these wounds, manifesting as difficulties in emotional regulation, low self-esteem, and a persistent feeling of not being worthy enough.

The shadows of childhood marked by narcissism can be projected on the quality of relationships, job performance, and the ability to face life's challenges. Adult children may find themselves dealing with repetitive cycles of negative self-evaluation and self-demand , stemming from childhood experiences rooted in maternal narcissism.

B) Difficulties in Interpersonal Relationships: Shadows that Darken Human Connection

Interpersonal relationships for adult children of narcissistic mothers can be challenging and complex terrain. Shadows of maternal narcissism can affect the ability to trust, set healthy boundaries, and fully experience intimacy.

The struggle to build strong emotional connections can be a constant in the lives of adult children. The shadows of maternal narcissism can be projected in their interactions, creating difficulties in forming authentic and satisfying relationships. Feeling vulnerable and constantly seeking validation can influence your ability to make meaningful connections.

C) Challenges in Professional and Personal Development: Shadows that Permeate the Life Path

The shadows of maternal narcissism can also permeate the professional and personal life path of adult children. Difficulties in building a solid identity and the persistent search for validation can affect professional development and personal goals.

Adult children may face challenges in making autonomous decisions and building a life that reflects their true desires and values. The shadows of maternal narcissism can act as obstacles, generating doubts and self-questioning in the search for self-actualization.

D) Relentless Self-Demand : The Echo of Unattainable Perfectionism

Unattainable perfectionism instilled during childhood under maternal narcissism can persist into adult life. Adult children may find themselves trapped in a cycle of relentless self-demand , where any deviation from unreasonable standards can trigger feelings of inadequacy.

This self-demand can affect the mental and emotional health of adult children, generating anxiety, stress and a constant feeling of not measuring up. The shadows of perfectionism instilled during childhood can be projected in all areas of life, from personal relationships to job performance.

Chapter 5: Coping Strategies

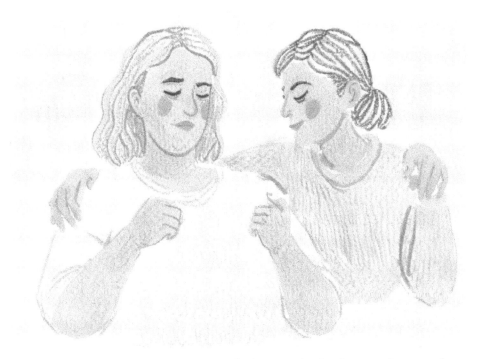

In the fifth chapter of our journey through the complex landscape of maternal narcissism, we will delve into coping strategies. This chapter is a guiding beacon, a compass for those who have navigated the stormy waters of having a narcissistic mother. Here, we will explore specific strategies designed to help children confront, manage, and ultimately heal from the aftereffects of maternal narcissism.

Coping strategies are not only a means to survive the storms of maternal narcissism, but also to flourish despite them. By exploring this chapter, children will find tools to reclaim their power, set boundaries that protect their emotional well-being, and build a strong foundation for healthy, authentic relationships. It is time to arm those who have experienced the shadows of maternal narcissism with the strategies that will help them navigate and conquer the stormy waters toward healing and personal growth.

5.1 Developing coping skills

Confronting the complexities of maternal narcissism is a monumental task that requires not only understanding but also a robust set of coping skills. This chapter is a guiding beacon that illuminates specific strategies designed to equip children with the tools necessary to navigate the storms and remain steadfast in the pursuit of healing.

1. Identification and Validation of Emotions: The First Line of Defense

Developing coping skills begins with recognizing and validating emotions. In an environment affected by maternal narcissism, children often face an avalanche of complex emotions, from frustration to sadness and anger. Learning to identify and validate these emotions is like establishing the first line of defense.

Recognizing that emotions are valid and understandable, even when they seem overwhelming or conflicting, is the first step toward building emotional resilience . Personal validation acts as an emotional anchor, providing stability amid the emotional storms that can arise in interactions with a narcissistic mother.

2. Establishing Healthy Boundaries: Protecting Emotional Wellbeing

One of the most essential coping skills in the context of maternal narcissism is setting healthy boundaries. This involves clearly defining what is acceptable and what is not in interactions with the narcissistic mother. Setting boundaries is not an act of confrontation, but rather a way to protect emotional well-being.

These boundaries may include effectively communicating personal needs, setting realistic expectations, and, when necessary, temporarily or permanently distancing yourself from interactions that are toxic. Developing the skill of setting healthy boundaries is like anchoring a boat in turbulent waters, providing stability and protection.

3. Promoting Self-Assertion: Building Internal Strength

Self-affirmation is a powerful tool in the arsenal of coping skills. In a narcissistic environment, where external validation can be scarce, learning to affirm yourself internally becomes a fundamental pillar for mental and emotional health.

Promoting self-affirmation involves recognizing and appreciating one's own achievements, qualities and worth. Children can cultivate an internal strength that acts as a shield against external invalidation. This includes challenging critical inner voices that may have been internalized during childhood and replacing them with messages of self-affirmation and self-love .

4. Developing Emotional Resilience : Learning from Storms

Emotional resilience is the ability to recover from adversity and learn from difficult experiences. Developing this skill involves seeing emotional storms as opportunities to grow and become stronger rather than weaker.

Children can learn to process and manage emotional pain, cultivating a resilient mindset that helps them face challenges with strength. Emotional resilience acts as a rudder that allows children to navigate stormy waters without losing sight of their ability to recover and grow despite difficulties.

5. Search for External Support: Redefining the Navigation Team

Developing coping skills does not mean facing storms alone. Seeking external support is a vital strategy. This may include participating in therapy, whether individual or group, or connecting with friends and loved ones who can provide solid support.

Building external support equipment is like strengthening the hull of a ship, providing additional stability and strength. Sharing experiences with others who have navigated similar waters can be comforting and provide valuable perspectives.

5.2 Setting healthy boundaries

Establishing healthy boundaries emerges as a fundamental tool to protect emotional well-being. This ability is like erecting an emotional fortress that guards against the tumultuous tides of manipulation and invalidation.

The Foundation of a Healthy Relationship: Limits on the Mother-Child Dynamic

Healthy boundaries are the foundation on which emotionally balanced relationships are built. In the context of mother-child dynamics, setting limits involves clearly defining what behaviors and interactions are acceptable and which are not. It is an act of emotional self-defense, an affirmation of one's own worth and dignity.

Children can set limits by clearly communicating their needs and expectations to the narcissistic mother. This may involve expressing firmly but respectfully how they wish to be treated and what behaviors they will not tolerate. Setting boundaries is not an act of confrontation, but rather an assertion of autonomy and the right to be treated with respect.

Recognizing the Signs of Boundary Violations: Red Alert in Relationships

A crucial part of setting healthy boundaries is recognizing the signs of boundary violations. The narcissistic mother may consciously or unconsciously challenge these boundaries, and children must be alert to warning signs. This may include derogatory comments, invasions of privacy, excessive demands for attention, or emotional manipulations.

Recognizing these signs is like raising a red flag in relationships. It allows children to identify situations in which their limits are being challenged and take steps to protect their emotional well-being.

Clear and Assertive Communication: The Sword and the Shield in Defending Limits

Clear and assertive communication is the sword and shield in defending healthy boundaries. Children can learn to express their needs directly and respectfully, without fear of retaliation or judgment. Assertiveness involves maintaining one's truth without aggression or submission.

Clear and assertive communication establishes a tone of mutual respect in interactions. Children can practice expressing boundaries in a positive way, focusing on their own needs and rights rather than accusations toward the narcissistic mother. This strengthens the position of the children and creates a basis for more equitable relationships.

Consistency in Boundary Application: Building Robust Borders

Consistency is the key to building robust boundaries. Setting boundaries is not a one-time event, but rather an ongoing process that requires perseverance and consistency. Children must remain firm in enforcing boundaries, even when faced with resistance or manipulation from the narcissistic mother.

Consistency in applying boundaries is like building a strong wall. Every time children defend their boundaries, they reinforce the integrity of their emotional well-being. This also sends a clear message to the narcissistic mother that boundaries are inviolable and that mutual respect is essential in the relationship.

Learning to Say "No": Empowerment in Denial

Saying "no" is an empowering act that is critical in establishing healthy boundaries. Children can learn to say "no" firmly and respectfully when faced with unfair demands or emotional manipulations. This is not only an affirmation of one's autonomy, but also a protection against exhaustion and invalidation.

Learning to say "no" involves recognizing your own limits and respecting yourself enough to defend them. It is a valuable tool for preserving emotional energy and maintaining a healthy connection with one's own truth and needs.

5.3 Seeking professional and therapeutic support

In the challenging journey of facing maternal narcissism, seeking professional and therapeutic support emerges as a guiding beacon, illuminating the path to healing. The vital importance of turning to experts who can offer specialized tools and valuable perspectives to help children confront and overcome the emotional consequences of maternal narcissism is highlighted.

1. Understanding the Role of the Practitioner: Partners in Healing

Specialized professionals and therapists play a crucial role in the journey toward healing. They act as expert partners who can provide deep understanding of the specific relational and emotional dynamics of maternal narcissism. Their experience becomes a valuable guide for children, offering strategies adapted to their individual needs.

Professionals can help children explore and process complex emotions, providing practical tools to address the specific challenges that arise in relationships affected by maternal narcissism. Their role goes beyond problem solving, encompassing creating a safe space for emotional expression and encouraging effective coping strategies.

2. The Power of Individual Therapy: Exploring the Inner World

Individual therapy emerges as a powerful tool to explore the inner world and address emotional wounds. In a safe and confidential environment, children can share their experiences, fears and aspirations with a therapist. This therapeutic dialogue acts as a mirror that reflects and validates emotions, providing an external perspective that enriches personal understanding.

Individual therapy also offers a space to develop personalized coping strategies and address patterns of thinking and behavior that may have become ingrained during childhood. By exploring the deeper layers of emotional experience, children can find clarity and direction on their path to healing.

3. Support Groups: The Strength of Shared Community

The strength of shared community shines in support groups. Connecting with others who have navigated similar waters provides a sense of belonging and mutual understanding. Support groups offer a space to share experiences, strategies and achievements, creating a support network that strengthens each member.

Participating in support groups can reduce emotional isolation, providing validation and empathy that is often missing in relationships affected by maternal narcissism. The shared community becomes a constant reminder that you are not alone in your journey, building a sense of unity and collective strength.

4. Family Therapy: Rebuilding Relational Bridges

Family therapy focuses on rebuilding relational bridges within the context of the family affected by maternal narcissism. This approach allows both the children and the narcissistic mother to participate in a therapeutic process designed to improve communication, foster mutual understanding, and establish new healthy dynamics.

Through family therapy, children can express their needs and concerns in a structured and guided way, while the narcissistic mother has the opportunity to understand how her actions impact others. This process, although challenging, can open the door to positive changes in family dynamics and promote collective healing.

5. The Importance of Consistency: Commitment to the Healing Process

Seeking professional and therapeutic support is an ongoing commitment to the healing process. Consistency in participation in therapeutic sessions and application of learned strategies is key to seeing sustainable results. Healing is not a destination, but a journey, and seeking professional support is an ongoing investment in emotional and relational well-being.

Chapter 6: The Road to Recovery

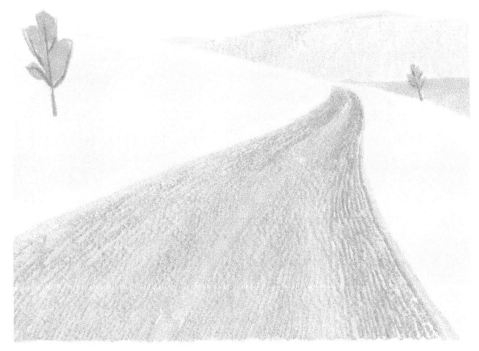

After exploring the different aspects of maternal narcissism and equipping ourselves with coping strategies, it is time to turn our attention towards recovery. This is not only a journey towards emotional healing, but also a journey of self-discovery and empowerment. Throughout this chapter, we will examine the practical steps and transformative insights that mark the path to recovery, offering children guidance in their quest for a healthier, more meaningful life.

6.1 Recognizing the need to heal

The first crucial step is to recognize the need to heal. This recognition not only involves being aware of emotional wounds, but also being willing to take the path to healing with courage and determination. In this segment, we will explore why recognizing this need is so vital and how this initial step marks the beginning of a meaningful transformation.

1. The Power of Self-Awareness: Looking Inside Yourself

Recognizing the need to heal begins with a powerful act of self-awareness. It involves looking inside oneself honestly and bravely, facing emotional scars and recognizing how past experiences have left an imprint on the psyche. This process of self-examination is not to point out blame, but to understand one's own history and its effects on current emotional health.

Self-awareness acts as a light that illuminates the dark areas of emotional experience. It allows children to identify patterns of thought, behavior and relationships that may be related to the influence of maternal narcissism. This self-analysis is the foundation on which the path to recovery is built.

2. Accept Emotional Reality: Validating Your Own Experiences

Accepting emotional reality is a fundamental step in the recognition process. Here, children validate their own emotional experiences, recognizing that their feelings and reactions are legitimate and understandable. It may involve letting go of self-blame and understanding that family dynamics, especially when they involve narcissistic mothers, can have a significant impact on emotional health.

Accepting emotional reality is like opening a door that allows understanding and empathy towards oneself to enter. This step is essential to free yourself from the burden of unfair blame and begin to address emotional wounds with compassion and patience.

3. The Value of Seeking Outside Help: Breaking Emotional Isolation

Recognizing the need to heal also means recognizing the value of seeking outside help. This can be in the form of trusted friends, supportive family members, or mental health professionals. Emotional isolation is common in situations related to maternal narcissism, and seeking outside help is a brave step to break that isolation.

Sharing your experiences with others who have been through similar situations can provide valuable perspective and a support network. Mental health professionals, such as therapists and counselors, can offer specialized guidance to address emotional complexities and provide effective tools for recovery.

4. Understanding Long-Term Impact: Motivation for Recovery

Recognizing the need to heal involves understanding the long-term impact of maternal narcissism on one's life. This understanding acts as a source of motivation for recovery. Understanding how past experiences can affect relationships, self-esteem, and overall well-being creates intrinsic motivation to work on one's own healing.

Understanding the long-term impact is also essential to challenging negative and self-demanding thought patterns that may have taken hold during childhood. Motivation for recovery arises from the vision of a future in which the influence of maternal narcissism no longer dictates quality of life.

5. Commitment to the Process: Building a Solid Foundation

Recognizing the need to heal culminates in commitment to the recovery process. This commitment is not just a one-time event, but an ongoing journey toward emotional improvement and building a more fulfilling life. It involves adopting a growth mindset, where every step, no matter how small, is a significant contribution toward recovery.

Committing to the process also means being willing to face challenges and celebrate achievements, no matter how modest. Recovery is a journey with ups and downs, but consistent commitment acts as the foundation on which to build a solid foundation for a healthier, more meaningful life.

self-acceptance process

It's about building a solid, independent and authentic identity. Let's delve into this process, exploring why it is crucial and how it can become a beacon of light on the path to healing.

Exploring Authenticity: Beyond Other People's Expectations

The process of self-discovery begins with exploring authenticity. Many times, in situations of maternal narcissism, children have grown up adapting to the expectations and demands of the narcissistic mother. In this process, it is common for them to lose sight of who they really are.

Exploring authenticity involves questioning the external narratives that have shaped identity. Children may begin to ask themselves: What values are really mine? What are my genuine interests and passions? This process not only helps to rediscover essential aspects of personality, but also allows us to build an identity based on authenticity and personal truth.

Accepting Complex Emotions: An Act of Self-Compassion

Self -acceptance , a key component in this process, involves accepting the complex emotions that have arisen as a result of the influence of maternal narcissism. This act of self-compassion recognizes that all emotions, even those that may seem uncomfortable or challenging, are valid and understandable.

Accepting complex emotions does not mean justifying the narcissistic mother's behavior or invalidating one's own suffering. Rather, it is about allowing yourself to feel, process, and release emotions in a healthy way. This act of self-compassion is like opening space for emotional healing and building a healthier relationship with yourself.

Discovering Personal Strengths: Building a Positive Foundation

The process of self-discovery also leads us to discover our own personal strengths. In an environment affected by maternal narcissism, children can often underestimate their abilities and qualities. Now is the time to explore and recognize these strengths as a foundation for building a more positive and empowered life.

Discovering personal strengths involves reflecting on achievements, overcoming challenges, and recognizing the unique abilities that each person possesses. It may be helpful to seek feedback from friends, mentors, or professionals to gain an outside perspective on individual strengths. This process is like building a solid foundation on which a stronger and more resilient identity can be built.

Defining Personal Goals: Driving Your Own Journey

On the path of self-discovery and self-acceptance , defining personal goals becomes a fundamental step. These goals should not be based on external expectations or the search for validation, but on what truly matters to each individual. They can be goals related to personal growth, emotional health, interpersonal relationships, or professional achievement.

Defining personal goals is like taking the helm of our own journey. It involves a commitment to continued growth and the pursuit of a meaningful life. These goals act as guiding beacons, illuminating the path toward a future built on authenticity and self-empowerment .

Cultivating Healthy Relationships: Building Authentic Connections

In the process of self-discovery and self-acceptance , the need to cultivate healthy relationships also arises. This involves establishing authentic connections with those who value and respect each individual's unique identity. It may require setting healthy boundaries with toxic people and fostering relationships that foster growth and positivity.

Cultivating healthy relationships is like planting seeds in an emotional garden. It requires care, attention and patience, but the authentic connections that flourish become a vital element in the recovery process. These relationships act as a support system that strengthens identity and contributes to emotional well-being.

6.3 Building healthy relationships

In the recovery process after facing maternal narcissism, building healthy relationships becomes an essential component. We will explore why these relationships are critical, how they can be built, and the transformative role they play in the journey to recovery.

A) The Importance of Healthy Relationships: An Emotional Haven

Healthy relationships act as an emotional refuge on the road to recovery. After tumultuous experiences with a narcissistic mother, building positive connections becomes a critical antidote to emotional toxicity. These relationships provide a safe space where children can experience love, support, and acceptance without judgment.

Healthy relationships are like a balm for emotional wounds. They provide a solid foundation from which children can rebuild their confidence in interpersonal relationships and develop a healthier understanding of human connection.

B) Establishing Healthy Boundaries: Protecting Emotional Wellbeing

In building healthy relationships, setting healthy boundaries emerges as a fundamental practice. After facing challenging dynamics with a narcissistic mother, children can learn to identify and communicate their needs clearly and respectfully. Setting boundaries protects emotional well-being and sets a tone of mutual respect in relationships.

Setting healthy boundaries is like building a protective fence around emotional health. It allows children to participate in relationships in an authentic and equitable way, avoiding the repetition of toxic patterns from the past.

C) Cultivating Positive Communication: The Key to Authentic Connections

Positive communication is the master key to building authentic connections. After facing manipulation and invalidation, children can learn to express their thoughts and emotions clearly and respectfully. Empathic listening and open expression create fertile ground for building strong relationships.

Cultivating positive communication is like watering the roots of a healthy plant. Strengthens the connection between people, fostering deep understanding and building emotional bridges.

D) Fostering Reciprocal Empathy: Building Bridges of Understanding

Reciprocal empathy is an essential component in building healthy relationships. After experiences with a narcissistic mother, children can appreciate the importance of understanding and being understood. Reciprocal empathy creates a bridge of connection, allowing both parties to feel seen, valued and accepted.

Fostering reciprocal empathy is like building a two-way street. Each person can move towards understanding the other, promoting a deeper and more meaningful connection.

E) Celebrating Individuality: Nurturing Diversity in Relationships

In healthy relationships, individuality is celebrated. After living under the shadow of the narcissistic mother, children can learn to value and respect the differences in others and in themselves. Celebrating individuality nurtures diversity in relationships, allowing each person to be authentic and appreciated for who they are.

Celebrating individuality is like blooming in a garden of unique varieties. Each relationship becomes unique and enriching, contributing to mutual growth.

F) The Role of Trust: Rebuilding Face-to-Face Connections

Trust is a key ingredient in building healthy relationships. After living with distrust due to maternal narcissism, children can learn to trust again. Trust is built over time through consistent actions, open communication and transparency.

Trust is like building a solid bridge. With every positive interaction, a brick is added, strengthening the connection and allowing relationships to flourish.

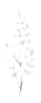

Chapter 7: Therapy and Support Resources

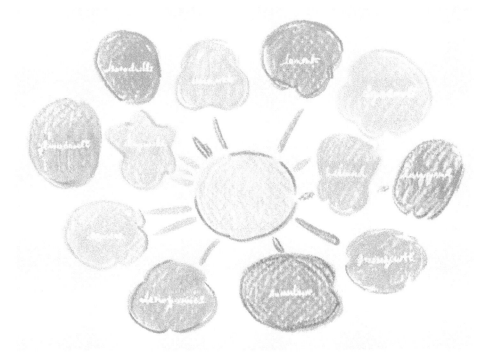

This chapter acts as a guiding beacon, illuminating the various tools that are available to those seeking to heal after facing maternal narcissism. We will explore specialized therapies, support groups, and other resources that offer guidance and support on the path to emotional recovery and personal growth.

7.1 Recommended types of therapy

On the path to healing after facing maternal narcissism, specialized therapies emerge as valuable and personalized tools that guide the recovery process. We will discover how these therapies offer specific approaches, providing meaningful support on the journey to recovery.

1. Talk Therapy: Unraveling the Emotional Narrative

Conversation therapy, also known as talk therapy , focuses on open dialogue and exploration of the individual's emotional narrative. In the context of the influence of maternal narcissism, this therapy provides a safe space for children to share their experiences, express repressed emotions, and explore the complexities of their relationships.

The talk therapist acts as a sympathetic guide, helping children unravel patterns of thought and behavior rooted in the influence of a narcissistic mother. Through verbal expression, a process of emotional release and construction of new, healthier narratives begins.

2. Cognitive-Behavioral Therapy: Challenging Negative Patterns

Cognitive behavioral therapy (CBT) focuses on identifying and changing patterns of negative thinking and behavior. In the context of maternal narcissism, this therapy addresses limiting beliefs and conditioned emotional responses. Children learn to recognize and challenge harmful patterns, replacing them with more realistic thoughts and healthy behaviors.

CBT provides practical tools to manage stress, anxiety, and self-esteem affected by narcissistic influence. By actively working to change negative patterns, children can experience a gradual transformation in their perception of themselves and the way they relate to others.

3. Schema Therapy: Addressing Deeply Rooted Beliefs

Schema therapy focuses on addressing deeply held beliefs that developed during childhood and continue to affect adult life. In situations of maternal narcissism, these beliefs can be distorted due to manipulation and invalidation. Schema therapy helps identify and change dysfunctional schemas, promoting greater self-awareness and authenticity.

By exploring the roots of thought and behavior patterns, children can better understand how narcissistic influence has shaped their internal schemas. Working on modifying these schemas allows for a deeper and more lasting transformation in their perception of themselves and the quality of their relationships.

4. Acceptance and Commitment Therapy: Living Fully

Acceptance and commitment therapy (ACT) focuses on accepting present experiences and committing to actions that are aligned with personal values.

In the context of maternal narcissism, ACT helps children accept complex emotions and engage in behaviors that promote emotional and relational health.

This therapy provides strategies to deal with emotional invalidation and manipulation, encouraging children to live fully and authentically. ACT focuses on building a meaningful life beyond the limitations imposed by narcissistic influence.

5. Group Therapy: Sharing Experiences and Strengthening Bonds

Group therapy offers an environment in which children can share their experiences with others who have faced similar situations. In the context of maternal narcissism, this therapy provides a sense of belonging and mutual understanding. Participants can share strategies, challenges and triumphs, building a valuable support network.

Group dynamics provide a safe space for emotional expression and validation of individual experiences. Group therapy acts as a constant reminder that you are not alone in your journey to recovery.

6. Family Therapy: Rebuilding Relational Bridges

Family therapy addresses relational dynamics within the family context affected by maternal narcissism. It engages the narcissistic mother and children in a therapeutic process designed to improve communication, foster mutual understanding, and establish new healthy dynamics.

Through family therapy, children can express their needs and concerns in a structured and guided way, while the narcissistic mother has the opportunity to understand how her actions impact others. This process can open the door to positive changes in family dynamics and promote collective healing.

7.2 Support groups and online communities

Support groups and online communities are presented as a virtual hug, providing a safe space where children can share experiences, find understanding, and receive valuable support. This segment explores the importance and usefulness of these groups, as well as how they form a network of meaningful connections on the road to recovery.

The Importance of Shared Connection: A Bridge of Understanding

A fundamental aspect of support groups and online communities is shared connection. Here, children find a bridge of understanding, since they share similar experiences related to maternal narcissism. This sense of connection eliminates the feeling of loneliness that often accompanies difficult situations, providing a space where every voice is validated and every story is understood.

The shared connection acts as a constant reminder that you are not alone on your journey. By joining a support group or online community, children experience a sense of belonging that contributes significantly to emotional healing.

The Strength of Validation: Recognition of Individual Experiences

In these virtual spaces, validation is a powerful force. Individual experiences are recognized and validated by those who have faced similar challenges. The narcissistic mother tends to invalidate her children's emotions and experiences, and these support groups offer a crucial counterbalance by providing an environment where every voice counts.

Validation acts as an empowerment tool. By feeling that their experiences are recognized and respected, children can begin to rebuild their confidence in themselves and the validity of their emotions.

Sharing Practical Tips and Strategies: An Exchange of Valuable Resources

Within these support groups and online communities, a valuable exchange of strategies and practical advice occurs. The children share approaches that they have found effective in dealing with specific situations related to maternal narcissism. From how to set healthy boundaries to how to handle difficult communication, this sharing of resources becomes a valuable toolbox for each individual.

This sharing of strategies not only provides practical solutions, but also fosters a sense of collaborative community. By learning from the experiences of others, children may feel better able to address the challenges that arise on their own path to healing.

Anonymity and Emotional Safety: Creating a Space of Trust

The online nature of these support groups and communities offers anonymity and emotional safety. Many children may feel reluctant to share their experiences in face-to-face settings for fear of judgment or retaliation. However, online, they feel free to express themselves without the fear of stigma or direct consequence.

This anonymity fosters a space of trust where children can open up without reservation. By feeling emotionally safe, they are more inclined to share intimate details of their experiences and seek the support needed to move forward on their healing journey.

An Empowerment Forum: Building Collective Resilience

These support groups and online communities act as empowering forums. Every story shared, every word of encouragement, and every valuable advice builds collective resilience . Children become sources of strength for each other, creating an environment where resilience is cultivated through connection and mutual support.

The empowerment forum becomes a beacon of light that guides each individual on their path to healing. Collective resilience is a transformative force that drives children to overcome adversity and move towards a fuller and more authentic life.

7.3 Resources for emotional recovery

After facing maternal narcissism, having specific resources can be like having a map to navigate tumultuous waters. This segment explores various resources designed to support emotional recovery, providing practical tools and strategies that guide the heart toward healing.

A) Self-Care Literature: Words that Embrace the Soul

Self-care literature is presented as a balm for the soul. Books that address topics of emotional healing, personal growth, and self-improvement can offer rich insights and practical advice. These works act as silent companions, providing comfort and direction in difficult times.

From self-help books to inspiring memoirs, self-care literature can be a valuable source of reflection and motivation. As children delve into these pages, they find words that embrace the soul and offer guidance on their journey toward emotional recovery.

B) Meditation and Mindfulness : Connecting with Inner Peace

Meditation and mindfulness are revealed as powerful practices to connect with inner peace. After facing the emotional turbulence of maternal narcissism, these techniques offer a space for calm and reflection. Meditation guides towards full attention, while mindfulness encourages awareness of the present moment.

Through these practices, children can learn to manage stress, calm their minds, and cultivate a more compassionate relationship with themselves. Meditation and mindfulness act as emotional anchors, providing a calm refuge in the midst of emotional storms.

C) Art Therapy: Expression without Words

Art therapy becomes a powerful form of expression without words. After facing maternal narcissism, children may find it challenging to put their complex emotions into words. Art therapy offers a creative means to express what is often ineffable.

From painting and drawing to creative writing and sculpture, art therapy allows children to shape their emotions in a way that goes beyond the limitations of language. This wordless expression becomes a therapeutic channel, releasing repressed emotions and encouraging self-exploration.

D) Mental Wellness Apps: Continuous Support in Your Pocket

In the digital age, mental well-being applications present themselves as continuous allies in your pocket. These apps offer a variety of resources, from guided meditations to mood tracking and breathing exercises. They are accessible tools that can be adapted to individual needs.

The portability of these applications allows children to access support anytime, anywhere. With features including self-care reminders and emotional journals, these apps become trusted companions on the journey toward emotional recovery.

E) Online Reading and Discussion Groups: Connecting with Virtual Communities

Online reading and discussion groups offer a unique way to connect with virtual communities. Through online platforms, children can participate in discussions about books related to emotional recovery and share their perspectives. This exchange with people who share similar interests creates a sense of community and belonging.

Participating in online reading and discussion groups expands the support network, providing the opportunity to learn from others' experiences and share knowledge. These virtual communities become spaces for mutual enrichment and support.

Chapter 8: Adult Mother-Child Relationships

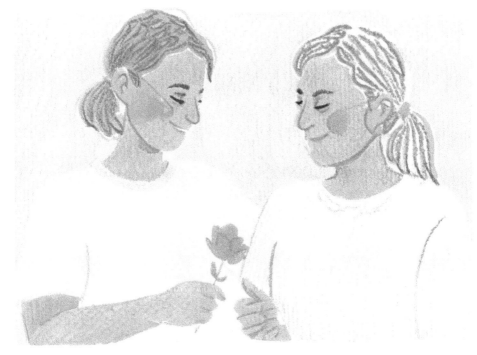

This segment shows us the transformative dynamic that arises when children, now adults, seek to establish mature and healthy connections with their narcissistic mothers. We will navigate the challenges, opportunities and strategies to build more equitable and authentic relationships in this new stage of life. Exploring these dynamics reveals the complexity of filial connection in adulthood and how healing can influence the course of these changing relationships.

8.1 Reconciliation or distancing

In the complexity of mother-child relationships in adulthood, the crossroads between reconciliation and distancing presents itself as a fundamental challenge. After years of narcissistic influence, adult children are faced with decisions that will significantly impact the quality of their maternal relationships. This segment explores the dynamics of reconciliation and estrangement, providing insights into how children can make informed decisions that reflect their personal needs and goals.

1. Reconciliation: Seeking a Path to Shared Healing

Reconciliation with a narcissistic mother involves finding a path to shared healing. This approach involves open dialogue and a willingness on both sides to address past wounds. Reconciliation is not an easy process, but for some children, it represents the hope of building a more authentic and equitable relationship.

Reconciliation can involve a mutual understanding of past experiences and a joint commitment to work toward building a healthier adult connection. It requires clear boundaries, open communication, and a shared effort to overcome the toxic patterns of the past.

2. Distancing: Protecting Emotional and Personal Health

Distancing, on the other hand, emerges as a strategy to protect emotional and personal health. After years of narcissistic dynamics, some adult children may find that distancing is necessary to preserve their well-being. Choosing distance doesn't necessarily mean cutting all ties, but it does mean setting clear boundaries to protect yourself from toxic influence.

Estrangement may be a valid option when reconciliation seems unlikely or when the relationship continues to be harmful to the adult child. Setting healthy boundaries and maintaining emotional distance can be essential to allowing children to focus on their own growth and healing.

3. The Difficulties of Reconciliation: Overcoming Communication Obstacles

Reconciliation, while noble in its quest for healing, is often marked by significant communication obstacles. The narcissistic mother may resist acknowledging her role in past dynamics and may have difficulty showing genuine empathy. Overcoming these obstacles requires patience, understanding, and sometimes the assistance of outside mediators, such as family therapists.

Lack of recognition by the narcissistic mother can lead to frustration in the adult child, making reconciliation a challenging process. Setting realistic expectations and working with a step-by-step approach can help overcome these difficulties.

4. The Risks of Distancing: Navigating Conflicting Emotions

Although distancing may be a necessary strategy, it also carries its own emotional risks. Adult children may experience feelings of guilt, sadness, and loss as they become estranged from their mothers. Social pressure and family expectations can also add additional emotional burden.

Navigating these competing emotions is crucial for the adult child to maintain their emotional well-being. Seeking support through friends, therapists, or support groups can help mitigate the emotional challenges associated with distancing.

5. The Role of Therapy in Decision Making

Therapy becomes a valuable tool in making decisions about reconciliation or distancing. A therapist can provide objective perspectives, help explore underlying emotions, and guide toward making informed decisions. Family therapy or individual therapy may be especially beneficial in addressing the specific dynamics of the mother-child relationship and offering strategies for building healthier connections.

The therapist acts as an impartial mediator, facilitating dialogue and helping both sides understand each other's perspectives. Therapy can be a safe space to explore options and make decisions critical to long-term emotional well-being.

8.2 Navigating the complexity of the adult relationship

The transition of the mother-child relationship from childhood to adulthood is a journey of self-discovery for both children and mothers. This segment examines the many layers that make up this complexity, from setting healthy boundaries to managing expectations, providing insights and strategies for navigating these emotional waters with wisdom and resilience .

Setting Healthy Boundaries: A Crucial Act of Self-Care

In adulthood, setting healthy boundaries becomes a crucial act of self-care. After years of narcissistic dynamics, adult children must learn to define and communicate boundaries that protect their emotional well-being. These boundaries act as healthy barriers that preserve emotional integrity and allow for more equitable relationships.

Setting boundaries may involve saying "no" to toxic behaviors, limiting the frequency of interaction, or clearly defining expectations. Although it can be challenging, learning to set boundaries is essential to building adult relationships that foster personal growth and emotional health.

Managing Expectations: Recognizing Changing Realities

Managing expectations becomes a key element when navigating the complexity of mother-child relationships in adulthood . Adult children often face the challenge of adjusting their expectations to the changing reality of the relationship. Recognizing that the narcissistic mother may not change radically is crucial to avoiding disappointment and frustration.

Managing expectations involves accepting the mother as she is, with all her limitations. This does not mean giving up hope for growth and change, but it does mean taking a realistic approach to building a relationship based on current realities.

Fostering Open Communication: A Bridge to Mutual Understanding

Open communication stands as a bridge to mutual understanding in the mother-child relationship in adulthood. Encouraging honest and respectful dialogue is essential to building a healthier adult connection. Adult children may strive to express their needs, emotions, and boundaries clearly and directly.

The narcissistic mother, in turn, can benefit from open communication that fosters empathy and understanding of her children's perspectives. Although it may require patience and effort, open communication becomes a fundamental means of building emotional bridges in the relationship.

Cultivating Reciprocal Empathy: An Essential Component for Connection

Reciprocal empathy is presented as an essential component for connection in the mother-child relationship in adulthood. Both children and mothers should strive to understand each other's experiences and emotions. Empathy creates fertile ground for emotional growth and building a more authentic connection.

Cultivating empathy involves putting yourself in another's shoes, recognizing and validating emotions, and striving to understand unique perspectives. This act of mutual understanding strengthens the foundation of the relationship and facilitates the building of emotional bridges.

Embracing Individuality: Recognizing the Authenticity of Each One

In adulthood, embracing individuality becomes essential to recognize the authenticity of each member of the mother-child relationship. Adult children must seek their identity independent of narcissistic influence and build a life that reflects their personal values and goals.

The narcissistic mother, in turn, must recognize and respect the individuality of her children, allowing them to grow and develop as unique beings. This process of embracing individuality contributes to building more equitable and respectful relationships.

Family Therapy: A Space for Joint Transformation

Family therapy is revealed as a valuable space for joint transformation in the mother-child relationship in adulthood. A family therapist can guide the process of building a healthier connection, providing tools and strategies to improve communication and manage conflict.

Family therapy also offers a neutral environment to explore family patterns, address underlying issues, and build bridges to a stronger relationship. Through therapy, family members can learn to understand each other better and work together toward common goals.

Chapter 9: Impact on Parenting

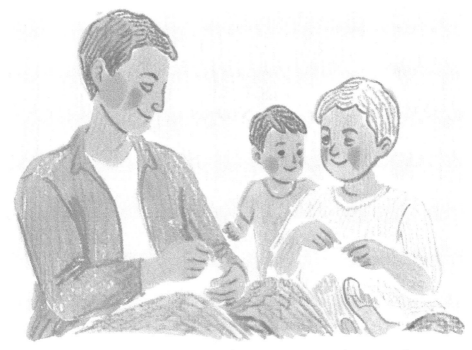

We will look at how experiences with a narcissistic mother can influence her children's ability to perform parenting roles and can affect how adult children approach raising their own children, examining the challenges and strategies for building mindful and healthy parenting. despite the shadows of the past.

9.1 How maternal narcissism affects parenting

In the complex fabric of parenting, the impact of maternal narcissism is revealed as a lingering shadow that can influence the way adult children approach raising their own children. This segment seeks to unravel the various ways in which experiences with a narcissistic mother can leave imprints on one's approach to parenting. We'll explore the specific challenges that may arise and how adult children, despite the shadows of the past, can cultivate mindful, healthy parenting.

Inheritances of Maternal Narcissism: Reproducing or Breaking Patterns

The inheritances of maternal narcissism manifest themselves in various ways in the upbringing of adult children. Some may find themselves unintentionally replicating the toxic patterns they experienced, while others consciously strive to break those destructive cycles. The influence of a narcissistic mother can affect adult children's perceptions of parenting , and confronting these influences is essential to building healthy relationships with your own children.

Challenges in Emotional Connection: Overcoming Inherited Distance

Maternal narcissism often affects adult children's ability to form strong emotional connections with their own children. The narcissistic mother's lack of empathy and focus on her own needs can leave adult children with difficulty understanding and responding to their children's emotional needs. Overcoming this inherited distance requires a conscious effort to develop emotional skills and foster a deeper connection with the next generation.

Balancing Self-Demand and Authenticity: Challenging Instilled Expectations

Self -demand and authenticity become areas of conflict for adult children who have experienced maternal narcissism. Some may feel an internal pressure to be "perfect" as parents, while others may struggle with authenticity, fearful of repeating the mistakes of their narcissistic mothers. Challenging these instilled expectations involves cultivating a balanced sense of self-demand that allows for personal growth and authenticity in parenting .

The Importance of Setting Healthy Boundaries: Protecting Family Dynamics

Establishing healthy boundaries becomes a vital tool to protect family dynamics. Adult children who have experienced maternal narcissism may face the challenge of setting effective boundaries with their own children while learning to respect their children's needs and boundaries. Implementing clear boundaries helps create a safe and equitable family environment.

Cultivating Open Communication: Breaking the Inherited Silence

Open communication is presented as a transformative force for adult children seeking to raise their children consciously. Breaking the silence inherited from maternal narcissism means promoting honest and respectful dialogue in the family. Adult children can learn to express their emotions in healthy ways and encourage emotional openness in their children, thus creating a space for mutual understanding.

Promoting Child Autonomy: Countering Overprotection

Overprotection is another shadow that can be cast in the upbringing of adult children who have experienced maternal narcissism. Promoting child autonomy becomes a key strategy to counteract this influence. Allowing children to develop independent skills and make age-appropriate decisions helps build a strong foundation for self-esteem and self-confidence.

Seeking External Support: Therapy and Parental Support Networks

Seeking outside support, whether through family therapy or parental support networks, is a valuable tool for adult children. Therapy can provide a space to specifically address inherited dynamics and offer strategies for mindful parenting. Additionally, being part of parenting support networks allows adult children to share experiences, get practical advice, and receive emotional support during their parenting journey.

9.2 Breaking the cycle in the next generation

Breaking the cycle of maternal narcissism in the next generation emerges as an act of courage and determination for adult children seeking to build a future free of shadows. From building solid emotional connections to promoting child autonomy, essential keys are explored to transcend the impact of maternal narcissism and build a bright family future.

1. Cultivating Strong Emotional Connections: Sowing the Seed of Unconditional Love

Cultivating solid emotional connections with children is presented as a fundamental tool to break the cycle of maternal narcissism. Through gestures of love, understanding, and emotional support, adult children can sow the seeds of unconditional love. This approach contrasts the lack of empathy experienced in childhood, thus creating an emotionally safe environment for their own children.

2. Promoting Child Autonomy: Building Foundations for Trust

Promoting child autonomy is essential to building solid foundations for children's self-confidence. By providing opportunities for independent decision-making and skill development, parents can counteract the overprotection associated with maternal narcissism. This approach encourages self-confidence and the construction of a positive self-image in children.

3. Promoting Open Communication: Opening Doors to Mutual Trust

The promotion of open communication stands as a door to mutual trust in the family. Adult children can create a space where emotional expression is welcomed and valued, thus breaking the silence imposed by maternal narcissism. Encouraging honest and respectful dialogue strengthens family bonds and lays the foundation for healthy relationships.

4. Challenging Parental Expectations: Creating an Alternative Model

Challenging parental expectations instilled by maternal narcissism involves creating an alternative parenting model. Adult children can work to move away from toxic patterns and adopt more equitable and respectful approaches. In doing so, they are building a different path for their own children, offering an alternative model of parenting that is based on understanding, respect and genuine love.

5. Building Family Resilience : Facing Challenges with United Strength

Building family resilience becomes a shield against the challenges that may arise when breaking the cycle of maternal narcissism. Adult children can recognize that mindful parenting will face challenges, but family resilience involves meeting those challenges with united strength. Collaboration and mutual support strengthen the family's ability to overcome adversity and build a healthier future.

6. Modeling Self-Care: Conveying the Importance of Emotional Health

Modeling self-care becomes a fundamental lesson for adult children seeking to build a healthy family future. By prioritizing their own emotional health and demonstrating self-care practices, they are instilling in their children the importance of taking care of themselves. This approach counteracts the lack of consideration for emotional needs that characterizes maternal narcissism.

7. Seeking External Support: Building Parental Support Networks

Seeking external support, whether through family therapy or parental support networks, strengthens efforts to break the cycle of maternal narcissism. Family therapy can provide a space to specifically address challenges and receive guidance in building mindful parenting . Being part of parenting support networks offers the opportunity to share experiences, get practical advice and receive encouragement during the journey.

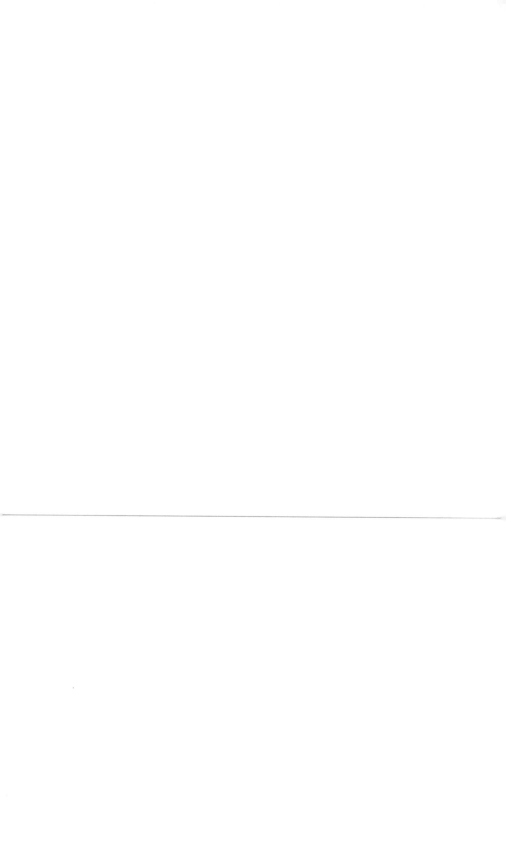

Chapter 10: Case Studies and Testimonials

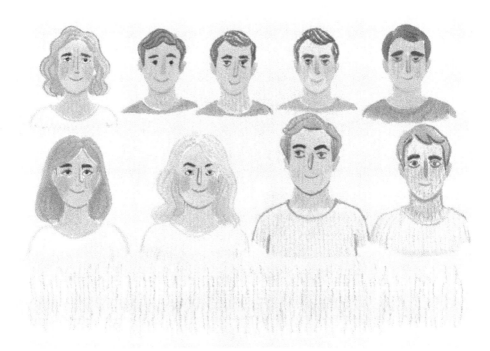

In the last chapter we have a space for narratives of resilience and transformation, where individuals share their experiences, challenges and, above all, their triumphs in the process of healing and building meaningful lives beyond the shadows of the past. These case studies and testimonials serve as beacons of hope and guidance for those seeking inspiration on their own journey toward emotional recovery.

These personal stories are living testaments to the human capacity to heal and grow, even in the most difficult shadows. Through these narratives, we seek to illuminate the unique paths each individual has traveled, offering inspiration and understanding for those seeking to understand and overcome the impact of having a narcissistic mother.

10.1 Narratives of Challenges and Triumphs

Each story presents its own set of challenges and triumphs, painting a vivid picture of the complexity of maternal narcissism and its consequences over time. From childhood marked by emotional invalidation to the search for identity in adulthood, these narratives explore the various stages of the journey to recovery.

A) Healing Wounds from the Past

The stories reveal how these individuals have dealt with the wounds of the past. Overcoming emotional manipulation, lack of empathy, and toxic patterns has required conscious effort and a commitment to self-care. Through seeking therapy, support from networks of friends and family, and the process of introspection, they have begun the journey toward healing.

B) Building Healthy Relationships

Building healthy relationships emerges as a recurring theme in these stories. The protagonists share how they have learned to set boundaries, encourage open communication, and foster strong emotional connections in their own families. These experiences highlight the ability to break destructive cycles and build a different relational future.

C) Lessons Learned and Advice for Others

In addition to their own journeys, these individuals share lessons learned and advice for those facing similar challenges. From the importance of seeking outside support to the need to cultivate self-care, these lessons offer practical guidance based on lived experiences.

D) Celebrating Personal Rebirth

Each story becomes a celebration of personal rebirth. These individuals have found the strength to transform pain into power, confusion into clarity, and adversity into opportunity for growth. Their stories inspire others to recognize the possibility of personal renewal and embrace the ability to build meaningful lives beyond the shadows of the past.

E) Promoting Community and Solidarity

These stories also emphasize the importance of community and solidarity in the recovery journey. Connecting with others who have experienced similar challenges provides a sense of belonging and understanding. Through support groups and online communities, these individuals have found a space to share, learn, and grow together.

10.2 The importance of sharing experiences

The powerful need and transformative impact of sharing experiences among those who have faced the challenge of having a narcissistic mother is imperative. The importance of opening spaces to tell real stories lies in creating a network of solidarity that provides support, understanding and guidance. This act of sharing experiences not only validates individual struggles, but also builds bridges toward collective healing.

Breaking the Silence: Liberation Through Expression

Sharing experiences becomes an act of breaking the silence that has often characterized the lives of those affected by maternal narcissism. Liberation through expression allows individuals to give voice to their experiences, facing the stigma and loneliness that often surrounds these topics. By sharing your stories, safe spaces are created where the truth can shine, providing a vital contrast to the emotional manipulation and invalidation experienced in the past.

Validation and Empathy: Building Meaningful Connections

The act of sharing experiences also provides validation and empathy. Those who have faced maternal narcissism find in the stories of others a reflection of their own struggles and triumphs. This emotional validation is essential for building meaningful connections, as it breaks the feeling of isolation and allows individuals to realize that they are not alone in their journey.

Mutual Learning: Lessons Drawn from Shared Experiences

The community formed around shared experiences becomes a space for mutual learning. Each story provides valuable lessons and practical strategies that others can apply in their own recovery journeys. From setting boundaries to fostering healthy relationships, shared experiences become a rich resource of collective wisdom.

Inspiration for Recovery: Beacons of Hope in the Darkness

Shared experiences act as beacons of hope in the darkness. Those who are at the beginning of their journey can find inspiration and strength in the stories of those who have made progress in their emotional recovery. This act of sharing offers insights into the possibility of personal renewal, showing that despite the shadows of the past, there is light on the horizon.

Building a Support Network: Strengthening Personal Bonds

The importance of sharing experiences lies in building a solid support network. Through personal connections, whether in local support groups or online communities, bonds are created that act as emotional anchors. These networks become valuable resources during difficult times, providing emotional support, practical advice, and the opportunity to grow alongside others who share similar experiences.

Conclusion

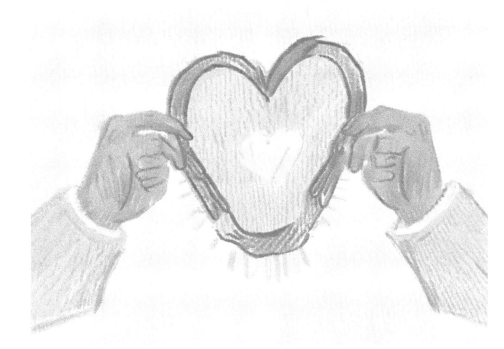

This book has not only sought to shed light on the dark reality of maternal narcissism, but also to offer guidance, support, and perspectives for those who have walked this complicated path. Each chapter has been a detailed exploration, using accessible words to understand and address specific aspects of this challenge.

Transformative recognition has been a key force. Validating individual experiences has been essential to breaking the silence, confronting emotional invalidation, and building a foundation for recovery. Every word shared has been an act of bravery, allowing voices to rise above manipulation and lack of empathy.

Through true stories, we have witnessed the unbreakable strength of human resilience . From childhood marked by confusion to the struggle to establish healthy boundaries in adulthood, each narrative has been a testament to the ability to heal and grow despite the shadows of the past. Resilience has been the driving force that has propelled the protagonists towards personal renewal.

The importance of sharing experiences has been fundamental in building a community of solidarity. Each shared story has contributed to a collective fabric of mutual understanding, joint learning and emotional support. These narratives have not only provided a mirror for those seeking their own truth, but have also built bridges to shared emotional recovery.

Throughout the chapters, we have charted the path to recovery. From recognizing toxic patterns to setting healthy boundaries, each practical strategy has been a tool for those seeking to transform their pain into power. The testimonies have been beacons of hope, guiding those who face the challenge of maternal narcissism towards a horizon of renewal and authenticity.

We not only reflect on the pages we have explored, but we look forward with the certainty that each word written has been a step towards healing, understanding and building a different future. May this book be a compass for those seeking light in the darkness, a guide on the journey to emotional recovery, and a reminder of the inherent strength that lies within each individual, ready to flourish even after the most difficult experiences. Facing the shadows of the past is the first step toward turning on the light on the path to a full and meaningful life.

Don't miss out!

Visit the website below and you can sign up to receive emails whenever Alexandria Publications publishes a new book. There's no charge and no obligation.

https://books2read.com/r/B-A-VDVCB-NADUC

BOOKS 2 READ

Connecting independent readers to independent writers.

Did you love *Narcissistic Mothers: The Truth about Being a Daughter of a Narcissistic Mother, and How to Overcome It. A Guide to Healing and Recovering from Narcissistic Abuse.*? Then you should read *Breaking Free from Narcissistic Manipulation: Strategies for Healing and Thriving Beyond Toxic Relationships*[1] by Olivia I. Thigpen (ENG)!

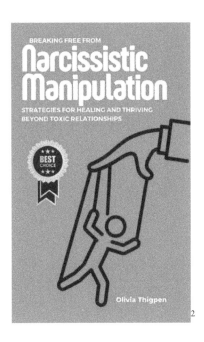

This transformative book will guide you through a journey of deep healing, helping you break free from the clutches of narcissistic relationships and flourish into a life filled with self-love and healthy relationships.

Immerse yourself in the pages of this book and learn to recognize the signs of toxic relationships, overcome low self-esteem, establish healthy boundaries, and cultivate empowering emotional resilience. With practical strategies backed by experience and expert knowledge, you will discover how to heal emotional wounds and build a life full of love, confidence, and positivity.

This book is much more than a self-discovery guide; is a beacon of hope for those who have suffered in manipulative relationships. Discover how

---

1. https://books2read.com/u/bzBQ62

2. https://books2read.com/u/bzBQ62

self-acceptance, self-care, and resilience can transform your life and lead you to genuine and fulfilling relationships.

Don't miss the opportunity to free yourself from the past, heal your wounds, and embrace a future full of self-love and meaningful connections.

Change your life today with "Break Free from Narcissistic Manipulation" and begin the journey to a new and better version of yourself!

Also by Alexandria Publications

Extreme Hypnosis for Rapid Weight Loss in Women: Learn How to Lose Weight with Hypnosis and Mental Power.
Learning to Manage Money: Financial Education from Childhood to Adolescence. Teaching Your Children to Save, Spend, and Invest Wisely
Narcissistic Fathers: The Challenge of Being a Son or Daughter of a Narcissistic Father, and How to Overcome It. A Guide to Healing and Recovering After Covert
Narcissistic Mothers: The Truth about Being a Daughter of a Narcissistic Mother, and How to Overcome It. A Guide to Healing and Recovering from Narcissistic Abuse.

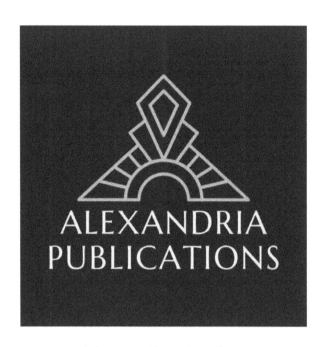

About the Author

At Alexandria Publications, we are dedicated to offering quality work supported by experts specialized in various topics. Our commitment to excellence is reflected in every book we publish. We collaborate closely with passionate authors to bring you a wide range of knowledge in various areas. Our mission is to provide you with valuable and enriching readings that feed your curiosity and inspire you to immerse yourself in the fascinating world of knowledge. Welcome to a constant journey of discovery!